Air Fryer

COOKBOOK

For Renal Diet

WHOLESOME AND DELICIOUS LOW SODIUM KIDNEY-FRIENDLY RECIPES FOR IMPROVED HEALTH

LINDA TERRENCE

Disclaimer

The recipes and information in this cookbook are for educational purposes only and not intended as medical advice. Please consult with your healthcare provider before making any changes to your diet or lifestyle. The author and publisher are not liable for any adverse effects or consequences resulting from the use of any recipes or information contained in this cookbook. The recipes are designed to be healthy, but individual nutritional needs may vary.

By using this cookbook, you agree to indemnify, defend, and hold harmless the author and publisher from any and all claims, damages, expenses, or liabilities.

TABLE OF CONTENTS

Introduction

Welcome to a world where health and flavor intertwine, where your diet journey meets the sizzle and pop of the air fryer!

Picture this: you stand in your kitchen, and the scent of anticipation fills the air as you gaze upon your trusty air fryer, ready to embark on a culinary exploration like no other. With each turn of the page, a symphony of flavors unfolds before your eyes, inviting you to indulge in a realm where taste and nourishment coexist harmoniously. How does that sound??

The **"Air Fryer Cookbook for Renal Diet"** is designed for individuals with kidney disease who want to make healthy and delicious meals using an air fryer. As a nutritionist with years of experience, I have seen firsthand the challenges individuals with renal disease face regarding food choices. That's why this cookbook provides a wide range of tasty and kidney-friendly recipes for breakfast, appetizers, main courses, side dishes, desserts, and beverages that can be easily prepared using an air fryer.

While following the renal diet can be challenging, air fryer cooking makes it easier to prepare healthy meals that are delicious and low in sodium, potassium, and phosphorus. Air fryers cook food with hot air. Thus, little to no oil is used. This makes it a perfect cooking method for individuals who are watching their fat intake and those who want to reduce the use of oil in their cooking.

Within these pages, you'll discover a treasure trove of recipes that not only satisfy your cravings but also honor the unique requirements of your renal diet. Every dish is meticulously crafted to delight your taste buds while supporting your renal health.

Unleash your creativity as you learn to adapt and customize recipes, transforming each dish into a unique masterpiece that suits your discerning taste.

Benefits of Air Fryer Cooking for Renal Diet

Air fryer cooking has gained popularity in recent years and for good reason. Not only is it a healthier cooking method, but it also offers many benefits for individuals following the renal diet. This section will explore some of the benefits of air fryer cooking for a renal diet.

Reduced Fat Intake

One of the primary benefits of air fryer cooking for a renal diet is that it allows for reduced fat intake. Traditional deep-frying methods require large amounts of oil, which can be high in saturated and trans fats. This can be problematic for individuals with kidney disease, as high-fat intake can contribute to other health problems such as heart disease and high cholesterol levels. Air fryers utilize the power of hot air to prepare food, minimizing or eliminating the need for excessive oil. Significantly fat intake is reduced, making it a healthier cooking option for individuals with renal disease.

Lower Sodium Content

Another benefit of air fryer cooking for renal diet is that it allows for lower sodium content in meals. Many pre-packaged frozen foods and snacks are high in sodium, which can be harmful to individuals with kidney disease. Air fryers allow individuals to prepare fresh, low-sodium meals at home, which can help to reduce sodium intake and support kidney function.

Retains Nutrients

Air fryer cooking also helps to retain the nutrients in food, which can be especially important for individuals with renal disease. The renal diet emphasizes the consumption of fresh fruits and vegetables, which are high in vitamins and minerals that support kidney function. Air fryers use hot air to cook food, which means that nutrients are retained in the food instead of being lost during the cooking process.

Quick and Convenient

Air fryer cooking is also quick and convenient, which can significantly benefit individuals with busy schedules. Many renal diet recipes require a lot of prep time and cooking time, which can be challenging for individuals with limited meal preparation time. This makes it a convenient cooking method for individuals who want to prepare healthy meals but only have a little time.

Breakfast Recipes

Air Fryer Omelet

Nutritional Info | Calories: 190, Carbohydrates: 11g, Protein: 10g, Fat: 12g, Sodium: 240mg, Sugar: 5g, Fiber: 2g

Prep Time: 15 minutes

Ingredients

2 large eggs

1/4 cup diced bell peppers

1/4 cup diced onions

1/4 cup chopped spinach

Salt and pepper to taste

Cooking spray

Instructions

1. Preheat the air fryer to 350°F.
2. In a bowl, mix the eggs and add salt and pepper together.
3. Proceed to spritz the air fryer basket with cooking spray.
4. Pour the egg mixture into the basket.
5. Add the diced vegetables on top of the eggs.
6. Cook the omelet in the air fryer for 5-7 minutes or until the eggs are fully cooked.
7. Use a spatula to remove the omelet from the basket carefully.
8. Serve hot, and enjoy!

Air Fryer French Toast

Nutritional Info | Calories: 220, Carbohydrates: 20g, Protein: 12g, Fat: 10g, Sodium: 270mg, Sugar: 3g, Fiber: 3g

Prep Time: 15 minutes

Ingredients

2 slices of whole-grain bread

2 eggs

1/4 cup milk

1/4 tsp cinnamon

Cooking spray

Instructions

1. Whisk together the eggs, milk, and cinnamon in a shallow bowl.
2. Preheat the air fryer to 350°F.
3. Spread the egg mixture evenly on both sides of each slice of bread.
4. Proceed to spritz the air fryer basket with cooking spray.
5. Place the bread in the basket and cook for 5-7 minutes or until the toast is golden brown.
6. Carefully remove the French toast from the air fryer with a spatula.
7. Top with your favorite toppings, such as maple syrup, fresh fruit, or whipped cream, and serve hot.

Air Fryer Breakfast Hash

Nutritional Info | Calories: 160, Carbohydrates: 22g, Protein: 2g, Fat: 8g, Sodium: 70mg, Sugar: 6g, Fiber: 4g

Prep Time: 20 minutes

Ingredients

1 large sweet potato, peeled and diced

1 small onion, diced

1 red bell pepper, diced

1 green bell pepper, diced

2 tbsp olive oil

1 tsp smoked paprika

1/2 tsp garlic powder

Salt and pepper, to taste

Instructions

1. In a large bowl, toss together the sweet potato, onion, and bell peppers with olive oil and spices until evenly coated.
2. Preheat the air fryer to 375°F.
3. Add the vegetable mixture to the air fryer basket and cook for 10-12 minutes or until the vegetables are tender and crispy.
4. Remove from the air fryer basket and serve hot with your choice of protein, such as eggs or turkey sausage.

Air Fryer Breakfast Sausage

Nutritional Info | Calories: 150, Carbohydrates: 0g, Protein: 8g, Fat: 12g, Sodium: 450mg, Sugar: 0g, Fiber: 0g

Prep Time: 15 minutes

Ingredients

4 breakfast sausage links

Instructions

1. Preheat the air fryer to 375°F.
2. Place the breakfast sausage links in the air fryer basket, ensuring they are not touching each other.
3. Cook the sausage links for 8-10 minutes or until they are fully cooked and browned.
4. Use tongs to remove the sausages from the air fryer basket and serve hot with your choice of sides.

Air Fryer Breakfast Burrito

Nutritional Info | Calories: 390, Carbohydrates: 28g, Protein: 28g, Fat: 20g, Sodium: 710mg, Sugar: 3g, Fiber: 6g

Prep Time: 15 minutes

Ingredients

2 whole-grain tortillas

4 eggs scrambled

4 slices of turkey bacon (chopped and cooked)

1 tomato, diced

1/2 cup shredded cheese

Instructions

1. Preheat the air fryer to 350°F.
2. Wrap scrambled eggs, cooked turkey bacon, diced tomatoes, and shredded cheese in a whole-grain tortilla.
3. Place the burrito in the air fryer basket and cook for 5-7 minutes or until the burrito is hot and crispy.
4. Use tongs to remove the burrito from the air fryer basket and serve it hot with your choice of sides.

Air Fryer Breakfast Frittata

Nutritional Info | Calories: 163, Carbohydrates: 3g, Protein: 14g, Fat: 11g, Sodium: 259mg, Sugar: 2g, Fiber: 1g

Prep Time: 20 minutes

Ingredients

6 eggs

1 zucchini, diced

1 tomato, diced

1/2 onion, diced

1/4 cup shredded cheese

Salt and pepper to taste

Instructions

1. In a mixing dish, whisk together the eggs and season with salt and pepper.
2. Add the diced vegetables to the eggs and mix well.
3. Proceed to spritz the air fryer basket with cooking spray and pour in the egg mixture.
4. Sprinkle shredded cheese over the top of the mixture.
5. Cook in the air fryer at 350°F for 10-12 minutes or until the frittata is set and lightly golden on top.
6. Use a spatula to remove the frittata from the basket and slice it into wedges to serve.

Air Fryer Banana Oatmeal Cups

Nutritional Info | Calories: 115, Carbohydrates: 26g, Protein: 3g, Fat: 1g, Sodium: 189mg, Sugar: 8g, Fiber: 3g

Prep Time: 20 minutes

Ingredients

2 ripe bananas, mashed

1 1/2 cups old-fashioned oats

1 teaspoon cinnamon

2 tablespoons honey

Non-stick cooking spray

Instructions

1. Preheat your air fryer to 350°F.
2. Mash the bananas in a large mixing basin until smooth.
3. Add in the oats, cinnamon, and honey, and mix until well combined.
4. Spray silicone muffin cups with non-stick cooking spray, and spoon the oatmeal mixture into each cup.
5. Place the muffin cups in the air fryer basket and cook for 10-12 minutes until the oatmeal cups are fully cooked and golden brown on top.
6. Once cooked, remove the muffin cups from the air fryer and let them cool for a few minutes before serving.

Air Fryer Breakfast Quiche

Nutritional Info | Calories: 237, Carbohydrates: 16g, Protein: 10g, Fat: 14g, Sodium: 283mg, Sugar: 5g, Fiber: 2g

Prep Time: 40 minutes

Ingredients

1 whole-grain pie crust

4 large eggs

1/2 cup milk

1/2 cup chopped spinach

1/2 cup shredded cheese

Salt and pepper to taste

Instructions

1. Preheat the air fryer to 350°F for a few minutes.
2. Roll out the whole-grain pie crust and place it in an air fryer basket. Press the edges to fit the basket.
3. In a mixing bowl, beat the eggs and add milk, chopped spinach, shredded cheese, salt, and pepper. Whisk until combined.
4. Spread the mixture evenly in the pie crust with a spatula.
5. Cook in the air fryer at 350°F for 20-25 minutes, or until the quiche is fully cooked and the crust is golden brown.
6. Remove the quiche from the air fryer and set aside for a few minutes to cool.
7. Cut the quiche into slices and serve warm.

Appetizers and Snacks

Recipes

Air Fryer Sweet Potato Chips

Nutritional Info | Calories: 150, Carbohydrates: 20g, Protein: 2g, Fat: 7g, Sodium: 90mg, Sugar: 10g, Fiber: 3g

Prep Time: 25 minutes

Ingredients

2 large sweet potatoes

2 tablespoons olive oil

1 teaspoon garlic powder

1 teaspoon smoked paprika

Salt and black pepper, to taste

Instructions

1. Preheat the air fryer to 375°F.
2. Wash and dry the sweet potatoes. Cut them into thin slices using a sharp knife or mandoline slicer.
3. Toss the sweet potato slices with olive oil, garlic powder, smoked paprika, salt, and black pepper in a bowl.
4. Place the sweet potato slices in the air fryer basket in a single layer, ensuring they don't overlap.
5. Cook the sweet potato chips for 8-10 minutes, flipping them halfway through the cooking time until they are crispy and golden brown.
6. Serve the chips immediately, and enjoy!

Air Fryer Chicken Wings

Nutritional Info | Calories: 240, Carbohydrates: 1g, Protein: 21g, Fat: 16g, Sodium: 250mg, Sugar: 0g, Fiber: 0g

Prep Time: 35 minutes

Ingredients

1 lb. chicken wings

1 tsp garlic powder

1 tsp paprika

1 tbsp olive oil

Salt and pepper, to taste

Instructions

1. Preheat the air fryer to 375°F for 3-5 minutes.
2. Mix the garlic powder, paprika, olive oil, salt, and pepper in a bowl.
3. Add the chicken wings to the bowl and coat them with the mixture.
4. Lay the chicken wings in a single layer in the air fryer basket.
5. Cook for 20-25 minutes, flipping halfway through.
6. Serve with your favorite dipping sauce.

Air Fryer Zucchini Fries

Nutritional Info | Calories: 124, Carbohydrates: 18g, Protein: 6g, Fat: 4g, Sodium: 397mg, Sugar: 11g, Fiber: 2g

Prep Time: 25 minutes

Ingredients

2 medium zucchinis, sliced into sticks

1/2 cup bread crumbs

1/4 cup grated Parmesan cheese

1/2 tsp garlic powder

1/4 tsp salt

1/4 tsp black pepper

1 egg

Cooking spray

Instructions

1. Beat the egg in a bowl, then put aside.
2. In another bowl, mix the bread crumbs, Parmesan cheese, garlic powder, salt, and black pepper.
3. Dip each zucchini stick in the beaten egg and coat it in the breadcrumb mixture.
4. Place the coated zucchini sticks in an air fryer basket, ensuring they do not touch each other.
5. Proceed to spritz the air fryer basket with cooking spray.
6. Cook in the air fryer at 375°F for 10-12 minutes, flipping halfway through the cooking time, until the fries are crispy and golden brown.
7. Serve hot with your favorite dipping sauce.

Air Fryer Turkey Meatballs

Nutritional Info | Calories: 194, Carbohydrates: 5g, Protein: 23g, Fat: 0g, Sodium: 423mg, Sugar: 1g, Fiber: 0g

Prep Time: 20 minutes

Ingredients

1 pound ground turkey

1/2 cup chopped onion

1 teaspoon minced garlic

1/2 cup breadcrumbs

1 egg

1 teaspoon salt

1/4 teaspoon black pepper

Cooking spray

Instructions

1. In a mixing bowl, combine the ground turkey, chopped onion, minced garlic, breadcrumbs, egg, salt, and black pepper. Mix well.
2. Form the mixture into small balls and place them in the air fryer basket, ensuring they are not touching.
3. Lightly spray the meatballs with cooking spray.
4. Air fry at 375°F for 10-12 minutes or until the meatballs are fully cooked and golden brown.
5. Serve hot with your favorite dipping sauce.

Air Fryer Stuffed Mushrooms

Nutritional Info | Calories: 60, Carbohydrates: 4g, Protein: 3g, Fat: 4g, Sodium: 148mg, Sugar: 1g, Fiber: 1g

Prep Time: 20 minutes

Ingredients

12 medium-sized mushrooms, cleaned and stems removed

4 oz cream cheese, softened

1/4 cup chopped spinach

1 garlic clove, minced

1/4 cup grated Parmesan cheese

1/4 tsp salt

1/4 tsp black pepper

Olive oil cooking spray

Instructions

1. In a bowl, mix the cream cheese, spinach, garlic, Parmesan cheese, salt, and black pepper until well combined.
2. Fill each mushroom cap halfway with the cream cheese mixture.
3. Preheat your air fryer to 375°F.
4. Proceed to spritz the air fryer basket with cooking spray.
5. Place the stuffed mushrooms in the basket.
6. Cook for 10-12 minutes or until the mushrooms are tender and the filling is hot and bubbly.

Air Fryer Eggplant Dip

Nutritional Info | Calories: 160, Carbohydrates: 7g, Protein: 2g, Fat: 9g, Sodium: 327mg, Sugar: 0g, Fiber: 3g

Prep Time: 30 minutes

Ingredients

1 medium eggplant, cut into cubes

2 tbsp olive oil

1 tsp salt

1 tsp ground cumin

1/2 tsp smoked paprika

1/4 tsp black pepper

2 tbsp tahini

2 tbsp lemon juice

2 cloves garlic, minced

Instructions

1. Preheat the air fryer to 375°F.
2. Toss the eggplant cubes with olive oil, salt, cumin, paprika, and black pepper in a bowl.
3. Place the seasoned eggplant cubes in the air fryer basket and cook for 15-20 minutes or until tender.
4. Once cooked, remove the eggplant from the air fryer and allow it to cool slightly.
5. Combine the cooked eggplant, tahini, lemon juice, and garlic in a blender or food processor. Blend the contents until it is smooth and creamy.
6. Serve the eggplant dip with pita chips or vegetables for dipping.

Air Fryer Kale Chips

Nutritional Info | Calories: 81, Carbohydrates: 8g, Protein: 3g, Fat: 5g, Sodium: 372mg, Sugar: 0g, Fiber: 2g

Prep Time: 15 minutes

Ingredients

1 bunch of kale

1 tablespoon olive oil

1/2 teaspoon garlic powder

1/2 teaspoon salt

1/4 teaspoon black pepper

Instructions

1. Preheat your air fryer to 375°F.
2. Wash and dry the kale leaves thoroughly. Tear the leaves into bite-sized pieces after removing the stems.
3. Toss the kale with olive oil, garlic powder, salt, and black pepper in a bowl until all the leaves are coated.
4. In the air fryer basket, arrange the kale in a single layer.
5. Cook for 8-10 minutes or until the kale chips are crispy and golden brown. To ensure consistent cooking, shake the basket halfway through.
6. Once done, remove the kale chips from the air fryer basket and transfer them to a serving dish.
7. Serve and enjoy as a healthy and tasty snack!

Main Course Recipes

Air Fryer Salmon

Nutritional Info | Calories: 265, Carbohydrates: 0g, Protein: 32g, Fat: 14g, Sodium: 384mg, Sugar: 0g, Fiber: 0g

Prep Time: 15 minutes

Ingredients

4 salmon fillets (about 6 ounces each)

1 tablespoon olive oil

Salt and pepper to taste

Lemon wedges for serving (optional)

Instructions

1. Preheat the air fryer to 400°F.
2. Brush the salmon fillets with olive oil and season with salt and pepper on both sides.
3. Place the salmon fillets, skin side down, in a single layer in the air fryer basket.
4. Cook for 8-10 minutes until the salmon is fully cooked and flakes easily with a fork.
5. Serve with lemon wedges, if desired.

Air Fryer Chicken Parmesan

Nutritional Info | Calories: 410, Carbohydrates: 19g, Protein: 49g, Fat: 14g, Sodium: 896mg, Sugar: 3g, Fiber: 2g

Prep Time: 45 minutes

Ingredients

4 boneless, skinless chicken breasts

1 cup breadcrumbs

1/2 cup grated Parmesan cheese

1 egg, beaten

1 cup marinara sauce

1 cup shredded mozzarella cheese

Salt and pepper, to taste

Olive oil cooking spray

Instructions

1. Preheat the air fryer to 375°F.
2. Combine the breadcrumbs and Parmesan cheese in a small mixing bowl.
3. Sprinkle salt and pepper on both sides of the chicken breasts.
4. Dip the chicken breasts in the beaten egg, then coat them in the breadcrumb mixture, pressing the crumbs into the chicken to help them adhere.
5. Spray the air fryer basket with cooking spray, then place the chicken in the basket, making sure not to overcrowd it.
6. Cook the chicken in the air fryer for 15-20 minutes or until the chicken is fully cooked and the coating is crispy and golden brown.
7. Remove the chicken from the air fryer and cover with marinara sauce and shredded mozzarella cheese on each breast.
8. Return the chicken to the air fryer for another 3-5 minutes, or until the cheese is melted.
9. Serve hot.

Air Fryer Stuffed Peppers

Nutritional Info | Calories: 300, Carbohydrates: 20g, Protein: 25g, Fat: 14g, Sodium: 430mg, Sugar: 6g, Fiber: 3g

Prep Time: 40 minutes

Ingredients

5 large bell peppers (tops cut off and seeded)

1 pound ground turkey

1 cup cooked brown rice

1/2 cup chopped onion

1/2 cup chopped mushrooms

1/2 cup chopped zucchini

1 garlic clove, minced

1 teaspoon dried oregano

1/2 teaspoon salt

1/4 teaspoon black pepper

1/2 cup shredded mozzarella cheese

Instructions

1. Preheat the air fryer to 375°F.
2. Mix the ground turkey, cooked rice, onion, mushrooms, zucchini, garlic, oregano, salt, and pepper in a large bowl.
3. Stuff the mixture evenly into the bell peppers.
4. Fill the air fryer basket with the stuffed peppers.
5. Cook for 20-25 minutes or until the peppers are tender and the filling is fully cooked.
6. Sprinkle the shredded mozzarella cheese on top of each filled pepper and cook for an additional 3-5 minutes, or until the cheese is melted.
7. Serve hot, and enjoy!

Air Fryer Turkey Burgers

Nutritional Info | Calories: 182, Carbohydrates: 6g, Protein: 22g, Fat: 9g, Sodium: 197mg, Sugar: 2g, Fiber: 1g

Prep Time: 20 minutes

Ingredients

1 lb. ground turkey

1/2 cup finely chopped onion

2 cloves garlic, minced

1/2 cup breadcrumbs

1 egg, beaten

Salt and pepper, to taste

Whole-grain buns

Toppings of your choice (lettuce, tomato, avocado, etc.)

Instructions

1. Mix the ground turkey, onion, garlic, breadcrumbs, egg, salt, and pepper in a large bowl.
2. Depending on the size required, shape the mixture into 4-6 patties.
3. Preheat the air fryer to 375°F.
4. Place the patties in the air fryer basket and cook for 10-12 minutes or until the internal temperature reaches 165°F.
5. Assemble the burgers on whole-grain buns with your favorite toppings.

Air Fryer Lemon Herb Chicken

Nutritional Info | Calories: 275, Carbohydrates: 2g, Protein: 16g, Fat: 0g, Sodium: 86mg, Sugar: 0g, Fiber: 0g

Prep Time: 35 minutes

Ingredients

4 boneless, skinless chicken breasts

1/4 cup olive oil

2 tablespoons lemon juice

2 cloves garlic, minced

1 tablespoon chopped fresh rosemary

1 tablespoon chopped fresh thyme

Salt and pepper to taste

Instructions

1. Preheat your air fryer to 375°F.
2. Whisk together the olive oil, lemon juice, garlic, rosemary, thyme, salt, and pepper in a bowl.
3. Coat the chicken breasts in the mixture.
4. Fill the air fryer basket with the chicken.
5. Cook for 20-25 minutes or until the chicken is fully cooked, flipping halfway through.
6. Before serving, allow a few minutes to let the chicken cool.

Dessert Recipes

Air Fryer Apple Chips

Nutritional Info | Calories: 62, Carbohydrates: 16g, Protein: 0g, Fat: 0g, Sodium: 1mg, Sugar: 0g, Fiber: 1g

Prep Time: 15 minutes

Ingredients

2-3 medium apples

1 tsp cinnamon

Cooking spray

Instructions

1. Preheat the air fryer to 375°F.
2. Wash and core the apples, then thinly slice them.
3. Spray the air fryer basket with cooking spray and place the apple slices in a single layer in the basket.
4. Sprinkle cinnamon over the apple slices.
5. Cook in the air fryer for 8-10 minutes, flipping the slices halfway through until they are crispy and golden brown.
6. Serve as a healthy snack or dessert.

Air Fryer Banana Oatmeal Cookies

Nutritional Info | Calories: 57, Carbohydrates: 12g, Protein: 1g, Fat: 1g, Sodium: 0mg, Sugar: 4g, Fiber: 2g

Prep Time: 20 minutes

Ingredients

2 ripe bananas

1 cup rolled oats

1/2 teaspoon cinnamon

Instructions

1. Preheat the air fryer to 350°F.
2. In a bowl, mash the ripe bananas with a fork until they are smooth.
3. Add the rolled oats and cinnamon to the bowl and mix well.
4. Pour the mixture into balls using a spoon or cookie scoop and place them on a baking sheet lined with parchment paper.
5. Place the baking sheet in the air fryer basket and cook for 10-12 minutes or until the cookies are lightly golden and set.
6. Remove the cookies from the air fryer and allow them to cool for a few minutes before serving.

Air Fryer Baked Apples

Nutritional Info | Calories: 153, Carbohydrates: 32g, Protein: 2g, Fat: 3g, Sodium: 30mg, Sugar: 1g, Fiber: 5g

Prep Time: 25 minutes

Ingredients

4 medium apples

1/2 cup old-fashioned oats

1 tsp cinnamon

1 tbsp honey

1 tbsp butter, melted

Instructions

1. Core the apples using an apple corer or a paring knife, leaving the bottom intact.
2. In a small bowl, mix the oats, cinnamon, honey, and melted butter.
3. Stuff each apple with the oat mixture.
4. Place the apples in the air fryer basket and cook at 375°F for 15-20 minutes or until the apples are soft and tender.
5. Serve warm, optionally, with a dollop of whipped cream or vanilla ice cream.

Air Fryer Blueberry Crisp

Nutritional Info | Calories: 210, Carbohydrates: 36g, Protein: 4g, Fat: 7g, Sodium: 2mg, Sugar: 22g, Fiber: 4g

Prep Time: 35 minutes

Ingredients

2 cups fresh blueberries

1/2 cup old-fashioned oats

1/2 cup almond flour

1 tsp ground cinnamon

1/4 cup honey

Instructions

1. Preheat the air fryer to 375°F.
2. In a mixing bowl, combine the blueberries, oats, almond flour, cinnamon, and honey. Mix well to combine.
3. Transfer the mixture to the air fryer basket.
4. Cook in the air fryer for 15-20 minutes or until the topping is crispy and the blueberries are bubbling.
5. Serve warm with a scoop of vanilla ice cream, if desired.

Air Fryer Chocolate Zucchini Bread

Nutritional Info | Calories: 115, Carbohydrates: 10g, Protein: 5g, Fat: 7g, Sodium: 6mg, Sugar: 4g, Fiber: 3g

Prep Time: 40 minutes

Ingredients

2 cups grated zucchini

3/4 cup almond flour

1/4 cup unsweetened cocoa powder

1/4 cup sweetener of your choice (e.g., honey, maple syrup, or stevia)

1 tsp baking powder

1 tsp vanilla extract

2 eggs

Instructions

1. Preheat your air fryer to 350°F.
2. In a mixing bowl, combine the grated zucchini, almond flour, cocoa powder, sweetener, and baking powder.
3. Beat the eggs in a separate bowl, then add them to the zucchini mixture.
4. Add the vanilla extract to the mixture and stir until everything is well combined.
5. Grease a small loaf pan with cooking spray or oil, and pour in the zucchini mixture.
6. Place the loaf pan in the air fryer basket and cook for 25-30 minutes or until the bread is fully cooked.
7. Remove the bread from the air fryer and set aside. Slice and serve when cool.

Air Fryer Peach Cobbler

Nutritional Info | Calories: 206, Carbohydrates: 38g, Protein: 4g, Fat: 6g, Sodium: 1mg, Sugar: 20g, Fiber: 5g

Prep Time: 40 minutes

Ingredients

4 cups sliced peaches

1 tsp cinnamon

1/4 cup sweetener of your choice (such as maple syrup or brown sugar)

1 cup oats

1/2 cup almond flour

2 tbsp honey

Instructions

1. Preheat the air fryer to 375°F.
2. In a bowl, mix together the sliced peaches, cinnamon, and sweetener of your choice.
3. In a separate bowl, mix together the oats, almond flour, and honey until well combined.
4. Place the peaches in the air fryer basket and sprinkle the oat mixture on top.
5. Cook in the air fryer for 20-25 minutes or until the cobbler is golden brown and the peaches are tender.
6. Serve warm, and enjoy!

Air Fryer Pumpkin Spice Donuts

Nutritional Info | Calories: 120, Carbohydrates: 7g, Protein: 5g, Fat: 9g, Sodium: 90mg, Sugar: 1g, Fiber: 3g

Prep Time: 45 minutes

Ingredients

1 cup pumpkin puree

1 cup almond flour

1/2 cup granulated sweetener of your choice

1 tsp cinnamon

1/2 tsp nutmeg

1/4 tsp cloves

1 tsp baking powder

1/4 tsp salt

2 large eggs

1/4 cup unsweetened almond milk

1 tsp vanilla extract

Instructions

1. In a mixing bowl, combine pumpkin puree, almond flour, sweetener, cinnamon, nutmeg, cloves, baking powder, and salt.

2. In a separate bowl, whisk together eggs, almond milk, and vanilla extract.

3. Pour the wet ingredients into the dry ingredients and mix until well combined.

4. Scoop the batter into a donut pan, filling each mold about 3/4 full.

5. Place the donut pan in the air fryer basket and cook at 350°F for 12-15 minutes, or until the donuts are lightly golden and a toothpick inserted into the center comes out clean.

6. Remove the donut pan from the air fryer and let the donuts cool for a few minutes before removing them from the pan.

Side Dish Recipes

Air Fryer Roasted Vegetables

Nutritional Info | Calories: 70, Carbohydrates: 8g, Protein: 2g, Fat: 4g, Sodium: 50mg, Sugar: 3g, Fiber: 3g

Prep Time: 20 minutes

Ingredients

2 cups of mixed vegetables (broccoli, cauliflower, bell peppers, carrots, etc.)

1 tablespoon of olive oil

1/2 teaspoon of garlic powder

Salt and pepper to taste

Instructions

1. Preheat your air fryer to 375°F.
2. Cut your choice of vegetables into bite-sized pieces.
3. In a bowl, toss the vegetables with olive oil, garlic powder, salt, and pepper.
4. Place the seasoned vegetables in the air fryer basket and cook for 10-12 minutes or until tender and lightly browned.
5. Shake the basket halfway through to achieve consistent cooking.
6. Serve hot as a side dish.

Air Fryer Garlic Green Beans

Nutritional Info | Calories: 31, Carbohydrates: 7g, Protein: 2g, Fat: 0g, Sodium: 16mg, Sugar: 3g, Fiber: 3g

Prep Time: 15 minutes

Ingredients

1 lb. fresh green beans, trimmed

1 tsp garlic powder

Salt and pepper to taste

Instructions

1. Preheat your air fryer to 375°F.
2. In a bowl, toss the green beans with garlic powder, salt, and pepper.
3. Arrange the green beans in the air fryer basket in a single layer.
4. Cook for 8-10 minutes or until tender and slightly browned, tossing halfway through cooking.
5. Serve hot as a side dish.

Air Fryer Cauliflower Rice

Nutritional Info | Calories: 48, Carbohydrates: 4g, Protein: 2g, Fat: 4g, Sodium: 107mg, Sugar: 0g, Fiber: 2g

Prep Time: 25 minutes

Ingredients

1 head cauliflower

1 tablespoon olive oil

1/2 teaspoon garlic powder

Salt and pepper to taste

Instructions

1. Wash and chop the cauliflower into tiny florets.
2. Proceed to pulse the cauliflower florets in a food processor until they resemble rice.
3. Toss the cauliflower rice with olive oil, garlic powder, salt, and pepper.
4. Preheat the air fryer to 375°F.
5. Fill the air fryer basket halfway with cauliflower rice.
6. Cook for 8-10 minutes, shaking the basket halfway through, until the cauliflower is tender and lightly browned.
7. Serve as a side dish or as a stir-fry or bowl base.

Air Fryer Garlic Roasted Broccoli

Nutritional Info | Calories: 80, Carbohydrates: 6g, Protein: 4g, Fat: 7g, Sodium: 120mg, Sugar: 0g, Fiber: 3g

Prep Time: 20 minutes

Ingredients

1 head of broccoli, cut into florets

2 cloves of garlic, minced

2 tablespoons of olive oil

Salt and pepper to taste

Instructions

1. Preheat the air fryer to 375°F.
2. Toss the broccoli florets in a bowl with the garlic, olive oil, salt, and pepper until equally coated.
3. Place the broccoli in the air fryer basket in a single layer, ensuring they are not overcrowded.
4. Cook for 8-10 minutes, shaking the basket halfway through, until the broccoli is tender and lightly charred.
5. Serve hot as a side dish.

Air Fryer Sweet Potato Fries

Nutritional Info | Calories: 118, Carbohydrates: 21g, Protein: 2g, Fat: 4g, Sodium: 311mg, Sugar: 1g, Fiber: 3g

Prep Time: 25 minutes

Ingredients

2 medium sweet potatoes

1 tbsp olive oil

1 tsp paprika

1/2 tsp salt

Instructions

1. Preheat the air fryer to 375°F.
2. Make long, thin strips out of the sweet potatoes.
3. In a bowl, toss the sweet potatoes with olive oil, paprika, and salt.
4. In a single layer, put the sweet potatoes in the air fryer basket.
5. Cook for 12-15 minutes, flipping once halfway through, or until the fries are crispy and golden brown.
6. Serve immediately.

Dear Reader,

Thank you from the bottom of my heart for journeying through the pages of "Air Fryer Cookbook for Renal Diet." I am truly grateful for your time, trust, and dedication in exploring this book's delicious possibilities.

In crafting this cookbook, I aimed to provide a valuable resource for individuals seeking flavorful meals while adhering to a renal diet. Your decision to use this cookbook demonstrates your commitment to your health and your willingness to embrace new culinary adventures.

By incorporating healthier cooking techniques, you've taken a significant stride toward achieving your wellness goals.

Remember, every recipe within these pages has been designed with your health in mind without sacrificing flavor or variety.

I hope this cookbook continues to be a source of enjoyment as you explore the vibrant and tantalizing flavors it offers.

If you have any questions or require additional assistance, please feel free to contact me at

lindahealthguide@gmail.com. I am here to support you on your path to a healthier, happier life.

I wish you a continued path of good health and culinary delight!

With sincere thanks,

Linda Terrence

Measurements Conversion

Volume

1 teaspoon (tsp) = 5 milliliters (ml)

1 tablespoon (tbsp) = 15 milliliters (ml)

1 fluid ounce (fl. oz) = 30 milliliters (ml)

1 cup (c) = 240 milliliters (ml)

Weight

1 ounce (oz) = 28 grams (g)

1 pound (lb.) = 16 ounces (oz) = 454 grams (g)

1 cup = 240 grams

1/2 cup = 120 grams

1/3 cup = 80 grams

1/4 cup = 60 grams

1 tablespoon = 15 grams

1 teaspoon = 5 grams

Please note that these conversions are approximate and may vary slightly depending on the ingredient and the density of the food being measured. It's always a good idea to double-check conversions and use a kitchen scale for precise measurements.

Temperature

$°F = (°C × 1.8) + 32$

$°C = (°F - 32) ÷ 1.8$

Linda Terrence

WEEKLY MEAL PLAN

	BREAKFAST	LUNCH	DINNER	SNACKS
SUNDAY				
MONDAY				
TUESDAY				
WEDNESDAY				
THURSDAY				
FRIDAY				
SATURDAY				

Linda Terrence

WEEKLY MEAL PLAN

	BREAKFAST	LUNCH	DINNER	SNACKS
SUNDAY				
MONDAY				
TUESDAY				
WEDNESDAY				
THURSDAY				
FRIDAY				
SATURDAY				

Linda Terrence

WEEKLY MEAL PLAN

	BREAKFAST	LUNCH	DINNER	SNACKS
SUNDAY				
MONDAY				
TUESDAY				
WEDNESDAY				
THURSDAY				
FRIDAY				
SATURDAY				

Linda Terrence

WEEKLY MEAL PLAN

	BREAKFAST	LUNCH	DINNER	SNACKS
SUNDAY				
MONDAY				
TUESDAY				
WEDNESDAY				
THURSDAY				
FRIDAY				
SATURDAY				

Linda Terrence

WEEKLY MEAL PLAN

	BREAKFAST	LUNCH	DINNER	SNACKS
SUNDAY				
MONDAY				
TUESDAY				
WEDNESDAY				
THURSDAY				
FRIDAY				
SATURDAY				

Linda Terrence

WEEKLY MEAL PLAN

	BREAKFAST	LUNCH	DINNER	SNACKS
SUNDAY				
MONDAY				
TUESDAY				
WEDNESDAY				
THURSDAY				
FRIDAY				
SATURDAY				

Linda Terrence

WEEKLY MEAL PLAN

	BREAKFAST	LUNCH	DINNER	SNACKS
SUNDAY				
MONDAY				
TUESDAY				
WEDNESDAY				
THURSDAY				
FRIDAY				
SATURDAY				

Linda Terrence

WEEKLY MEAL PLAN

	BREAKFAST	LUNCH	DINNER	SNACKS
SUNDAY				
MONDAY				
TUESDAY				
WEDNESDAY				
THURSDAY				
FRIDAY				
SATURDAY				

Printed in Great Britain
by Amazon

30105083R00031